DYSPHAGIA COOKBOOK FOR SENIORS

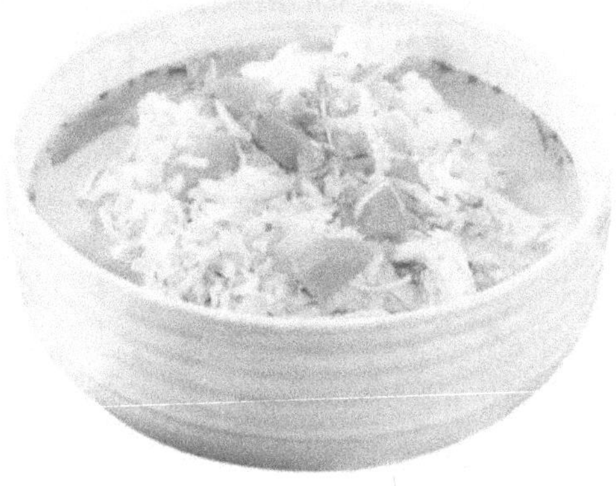

Delicious Recipes for Seniors with Dysphagia

Linda Carlucci

Copyright © 2024 by Linda Carlucci

DISCLAIMER

This cookbook is intended to provide general information and recipes.

The recipes provided in this cookbook are not intended to replace or be a substitute for medical advice from a physician.

The reader should consult a healthcare professional for any specific medical advice, diagnosis or treatment.

Any specific dietary advice provided in this cookbook is not intended to replace or be a substitute for medical advice from a physician.

The author is not responsible or liable for any adverse effects experienced by readers of this cookbook as a result of following the recipes or dietary advice provided.

The author makes no representations or warranties of any kind (express or implied) as to the accuracy, completeness, reliability or suitability of the recipes provided in this cookbook.

The author disclaims any and all liability for any damages arising out of the use or misuse of the recipes provided in this cookbook. The reader must also take care to ensure that the recipes provided in this cookbook are prepared and cooked safely.

The recipes provided in this cookbook are for informational purposes only and should not be used as a substitute for professional medical advice, diagnosis or treatment.

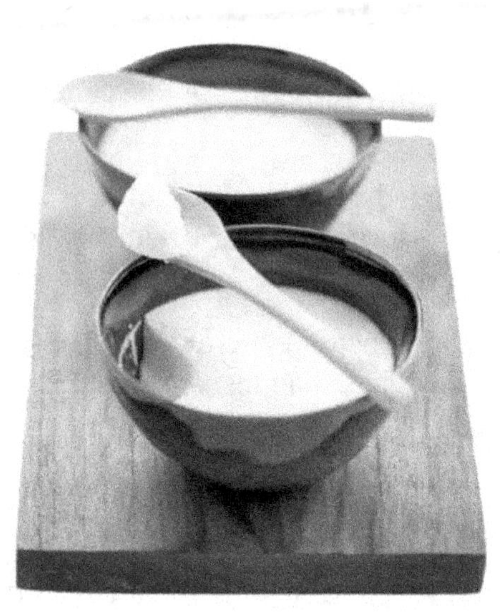

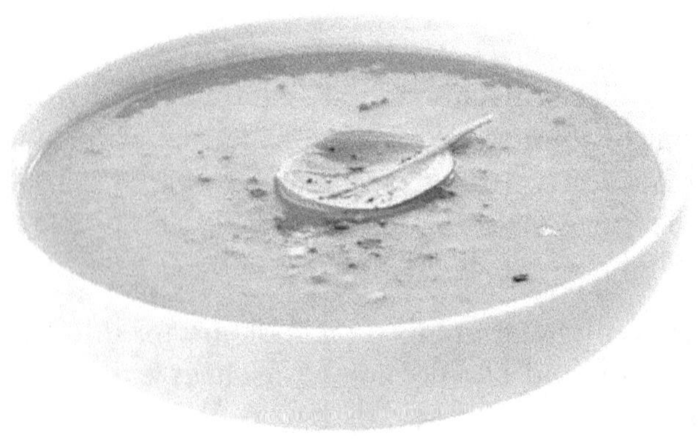

TABLE OF CONTENTS

INTRODUCTION

Dysphagia is a common condition among seniors which causes difficulty in swallowing. While it can affect people of all ages, seniors are particularly susceptible due to age-related changes in the swallowing mechanism.

This guide is designed to offer you a thorough comprehension of dysphagia, encompassing its causes, symptoms, diagnosis, available treatment options, and practical strategies for managing the condition.

Causes of dysphagia in seniors vary but often include neurological disorders such as stroke, Parkinson's disease, or dementia, which can impair the coordination of swallowing muscles.

Additionally, age-related changes in the throat muscles and decreased saliva production can contribute to swallowing difficulties.

Symptoms of dysphagia may include coughing or choking while eating or drinking, feeling as if food is stuck in the throat, regurgitation, unintended weight loss, or recurrent pneumonia due to food or liquid entering the lungs. It is crucial for seniors to recognize these symptoms and seek medical evaluation promptly.

Diagnosis typically involves a thorough medical history, physical examination, and various tests such as a swallowing study or endoscopy to assess the swallowing function and identify any underlying causes.

Treatment options for dysphagia may include dietary modifications, such as altering food texture or thickness to make swallowing easier, swallowing therapy with a speech-language pathologist to improve swallowing function, medications to reduce esophageal inflammation or treat underlying conditions, or in severe cases, surgical interventions.

Managing dysphagia requires a multidisciplinary approach involving healthcare professionals such as physicians, speech-language pathologists, dietitians, and occupational therapists. Seniors with dysphagia can also benefit from practical strategies such as eating slowly, taking smaller bites, chewing thoroughly, sitting upright while eating, and avoiding distractions during meals to minimize the risk of choking or aspiration.

CHAPTER 1

TYPES OF DYSPHAGIA

1. **Oropharyngeal Dysphagia:** This type of dysphagia occurs when there's difficulty moving food or liquid from the mouth into the throat (pharynx). It can be caused by neurological conditions like stroke, Parkinson's disease, or muscular disorders affecting the throat muscles.

2. **Esophageal Dysphagia:** Esophageal dysphagia refers to difficulty swallowing as food or liquid moves through the esophagus, the tube that connects the throat to the stomach. It can result from various conditions such as gastroesophageal reflux disease (GERD), esophageal strictures, tumors, or motility disorders like achalasia.

3. **Functional Dysphagia:** Functional dysphagia occurs when there's no apparent structural or neurological cause for the swallowing difficulty. It may be related to psychological factors, sensory processing issues, or behavioral patterns affecting swallowing function.

4. **Neurological Dysphagia:** This type of dysphagia is associated with neurological conditions that affect the nerves and muscles involved in swallowing. It includes oropharyngeal dysphagia caused by conditions like stroke, Parkinson's disease, multiple sclerosis, or amyotrophic lateral sclerosis (ALS).

5. **Structural Dysphagia:** Structural dysphagia arises from physical obstructions or abnormalities in the swallowing tract, such as tumors, strictures, diverticula, or anatomical abnormalities.

6. **Post-operative Dysphagia:** Some individuals may experience difficulty swallowing following surgical procedures involving the head, neck, or upper digestive tract. Post-operative dysphagia can be temporary or permanent depending on the extent of surgical intervention and individual factors.

COMMON CAUSES OF DYSPHAGIA

1. **Stroke:** Damage to the brain caused by a stroke can affect the nerves and muscles involved in swallowing, leading to dysphagia.

2. **Neurological Disorders:** Conditions such as Parkinson's disease, multiple sclerosis, ALS (amyotrophic lateral sclerosis), and muscular dystrophy can impair the coordination of muscles involved in swallowing.

3. **Gastroesophageal Reflux Disease (GERD):** Chronic acid reflux can lead to inflammation and narrowing of the esophagus, causing difficulty in swallowing.

4. **Esophageal Strictures:** Narrowing of the esophagus due to scar tissue, often caused by chronic GERD, can result in dysphagia.

5. **Esophageal Tumors:** Benign or malignant growths in the esophagus can obstruct the passage of food and liquids, leading to swallowing difficulties.

6. **Achalasia:** This rare disorder occurs when the lower esophageal sphincter fails to relax properly, causing difficulty in moving food into the stomach.

7. **Hiatal Hernia:** A condition where part of the stomach protrudes into the chest cavity through the diaphragm, potentially causing dysphagia.

8. **Pharyngeal or Esophageal Spasms:** Uncontrolled contractions of the muscles in the throat or esophagus can lead to difficulty swallowing.

9. **Zenker's Diverticulum:** A pouch that forms in the wall of the throat, which can trap food and cause swallowing problems.

10. **Muscle Weakness:** Weakness in the muscles of the mouth, throat, or esophagus due to aging, malnutrition, or neuromuscular disorders can result in dysphagia.

11. **Medication Side Effects:** Certain medications, especially those that cause dry mouth or muscle weakness, can contribute to swallowing difficulties.

12. **Radiation Therapy:** Treatment for head and neck cancers involving radiation therapy can damage the tissues in the throat, leading to dysphagia.

13. **Scleroderma:** This autoimmune condition can cause the tightening and hardening of tissues in the esophagus, resulting in swallowing problems.

14. **Eosinophilic Esophagitis:** Inflammation of the esophagus due to an allergic reaction, which can cause narrowing and difficulty swallowing.

15. **Poor Dental Health:** Missing teeth, ill-fitting dentures, or oral infections can make chewing and swallowing difficult, leading to dysphagia.

THE ROLES OF DIET IN MANAGING DYSPHAGIA

1. **Texture Modification:** Adjusting the texture of food to make it easier to swallow is crucial. Soft or pureed foods are often recommended for individuals with dysphagia to minimize the risk of choking or aspiration.

2. **Thickened Liquids:** Thickening liquids to a consistency that is easier to control and swallow can help prevent aspiration in individuals with swallowing difficulties.

3. **Avoidance of Hard or Crunchy Foods:** Foods that are hard, crunchy, or difficult to break down should be avoided as they can pose a choking hazard for individuals with dysphagia.

4. **Small, Frequent Meals:** Consuming smaller, more frequent meals throughout the day can help prevent

fatigue and reduce the risk of aspiration associated with larger meals.

5. **Slow Eating:** Encouraging individuals with dysphagia to eat slowly and take their time can improve swallowing safety and reduce the risk of choking.

6. **Chewing and Swallowing Techniques:** Teaching proper chewing and swallowing techniques, such as taking small bites, chewing thoroughly, and swallowing with the chin tucked, can improve swallowing function.

7. **Balanced Nutrition:** Ensuring that individuals with dysphagia receive adequate nutrition is essential. This may involve incorporating nutrient-dense foods into their diet to meet their nutritional needs despite dietary restrictions.

8. **Hydration:** Adequate hydration is important for individuals with dysphagia. Offering thickened fluids or providing hydration through alternative methods such as gelatin or ice chips can help maintain hydration levels.

9. **Monitoring Food Temperature:** Foods and liquids should be served at a safe temperature to prevent burns and discomfort, especially for individuals with reduced sensation in the mouth and throat.

10. **Avoidance of Alcohol and Carbonated Beverages:** Alcoholic beverages and carbonated drinks can exacerbate swallowing difficulties and should be avoided.

11. **Dietitian Guidance:** Working with a registered dietitian who specializes in dysphagia management can help develop personalized meal plans and ensure nutritional adequacy while accommodating swallowing difficulties.

12. **Incorporating Fortified Foods:** Fortified foods and supplements may be necessary to ensure individuals with dysphagia receive adequate vitamins, minerals, and calories.

13. **Maintaining Oral Health:** Good oral hygiene and regular dental care are essential for individuals with dysphagia to prevent oral infections and maintain oral health.

14. **Assistive Devices:** Using assistive devices such as adapted utensils, straws, or specialized cups can facilitate eating and drinking for individuals with dysphagia.

15. **Patient Education:** Educating individuals with dysphagia and their caregivers about safe swallowing practices, dietary modifications, and signs of aspiration can empower them to manage dysphagia effectively and prevent complications.

SIMPLE TECHNIQUES TO EASY SWALLOWING FOR PEOPLE WITH DYSPHAGIA

1. **Sit Upright:** Sitting upright while eating or drinking can help facilitate the passage of food and liquids through the throat and esophagus, reducing the risk of aspiration.

2. **Chin Tuck:** Tucking the chin towards the chest when swallowing can help close off the airway and prevent food or liquid from entering the lungs.

3. **Take Small Bites:** Encourage individuals with dysphagia to take smaller, more manageable bites of

food to reduce the risk of choking and improve control over swallowing.

4. **Chew Thoroughly:** Properly chewing food into smaller, more uniform pieces can make it easier to swallow and reduce the likelihood of food getting stuck in the throat.

5. **Swallow Twice:** After chewing food thoroughly, swallowing twice (once to move the food to the back of the mouth and again to propel it down the throat) can improve swallowing safety.

6. **Alternate Food and Sips of Liquid:** Alternating between bites of food and sips of liquid can help wash down food and make swallowing easier for individuals with dysphagia.

7. **Use Gravity:** Tilting the head slightly forward while swallowing can help gravity assist in moving food and liquids down the throat more smoothly.

8. **Swallowing Exercises:** Practicing swallowing exercises prescribed by a speech-language pathologist can strengthen swallowing muscles and improve coordination.

9. **Stay Relaxed:** Encouraging relaxation and reducing stress during mealtimes can help prevent tension in the throat muscles and facilitate easier swallowing.

10. **Modify Food Texture:** Adjusting the texture of food to make it softer, smoother, or more easily chewed can make swallowing safer and more comfortable.

11. **Thicken Liquids:** Thickening liquids to a consistency that is easier to control and swallow can help prevent aspiration and reduce the risk of choking.

12. **Use Straw or Syringe:** Drinking through a straw or using a syringe to deliver small amounts of liquid directly to the back of the mouth can help control the flow of fluid and improve swallowing safety.

13. **Take Breaks Between Bites:** Pausing between bites of food allows individuals with dysphagia to rest and regroup, reducing the likelihood of fatigue and improving swallowing effectiveness.

14. **Distracted-Free Environment:** Minimize distractions during meals to help individuals focus on chewing and swallowing without interruption, reducing the risk of choking.

15. **Monitor Food Temperature:** Serving food and liquids at a safe temperature can prevent burns and discomfort, ensuring a more pleasant swallowing experience for individuals with dysphagia.

FOODS TO AVOID FOR PEOPLE WITH DYSPHAGIA

1. **Hard Candy:** Hard candies pose a choking hazard and can be difficult to swallow, especially for individuals with swallowing difficulties.
2. **Whole Nuts and Seeds:** Whole nuts and seeds are hard and can easily become lodged in the throat, increasing the risk of choking and aspiration.
3. **Chunky Peanut Butter:** Chunky peanut butter contains large pieces of nuts that can be challenging to swallow. Opt. for smooth peanut butter or alternative nut butters instead.
4. **Popcorn:** Popcorn kernels can get stuck in the throat and pose a choking risk, particularly for individuals with dysphagia.
5. **Tough Meats:** Tough cuts of meat, such as steak or pork chops, can be difficult to chew and swallow,

especially for individuals with weakened swallowing muscles.

6. **Dry Bread or Crackers:** Dry bread or crackers can be hard to swallow and may cause discomfort or difficulty in individuals with dysphagia. Opt. for moist or soft bread alternatives.

7. **Raw Vegetables:** Raw vegetables, such as carrots, celery, or broccoli, can be difficult to chew and may pose a choking risk. Cook or steam vegetables until they are soft and easily mashed.

8. **Whole Grains:** Whole grains, such as brown rice or quinoa, can be challenging to swallow due to their coarse texture. Choose refined grains or finely ground grains instead.

9. **Large Pieces of Fruit:** Large pieces of fruit, such as apples or grapes, can be difficult to swallow and may pose a choking hazard. Cut fruit into small, bite-sized pieces or opt for softer varieties.

10. **Tough Skins or Peels:** Foods with tough skins or peels, such as sausages or hot dogs, can be difficult to chew and swallow. Remove the skin or peel before eating or choose alternatives with softer textures.

11. **Sticky Foods:** Sticky foods, such as caramel or taffy, can adhere to the throat and increase the risk of choking or aspiration. Avoid sticky candies and desserts.

12. **Spicy Foods:** Spicy foods can irritate the throat and esophagus, making swallowing uncomfortable for individuals with dysphagia. Opt. for milder seasoning and avoid spicy sauces or seasonings.

13. **Carbonated Beverages:** Carbonated beverages can cause gas and bloating, which may exacerbate swallowing difficulties and increase the risk of aspiration.

14. **Alcoholic Beverages:** Alcoholic beverages can impair coordination and increase the risk of choking and aspiration, particularly in individuals with dysphagia. Avoid alcohol or consume in moderation under supervision.

15. **Ice Cubes:** Ice cubes can pose a choking hazard and may be difficult to swallow, especially for individuals with dysphagia. Avoid chewing on ice cubes or using them to cool beverages.

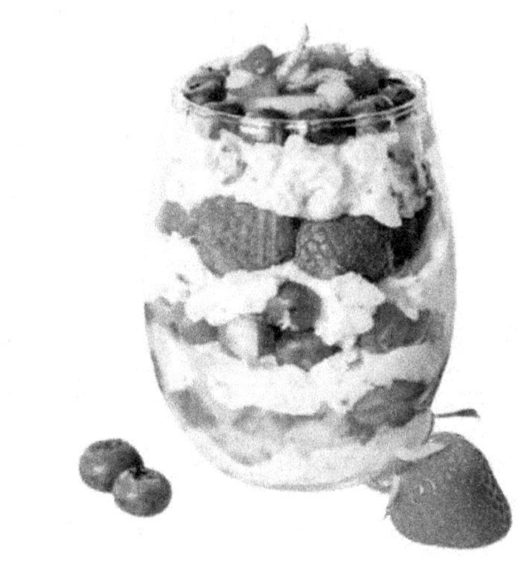

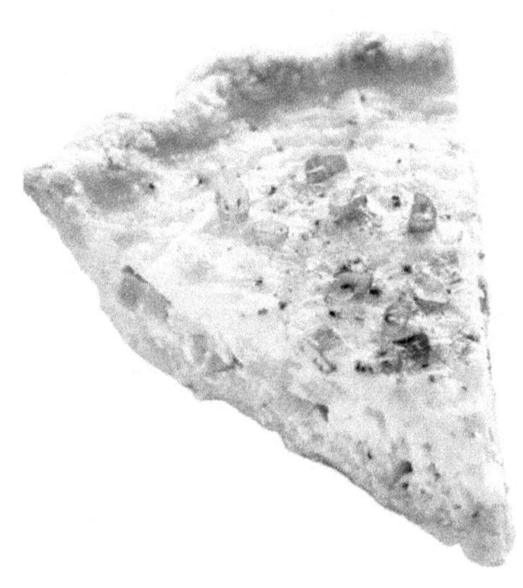

CHAPTER 2

14-DAY MEAL PLAN

DAY 1

Breakfast: Soft Pureed Vegetable Lasagna

Lunch: Creamy Cauliflower and Cheese Soup with Minced Chicken

Dinner: Soft-Cooked Pasta with Tomato Sauce

DAY 2

Breakfast: Pureed Chicken and Vegetable Soup

Lunch: Minced Shrimp Risotto

Dinner: Creamy Chicken and Rice Casserole

DAY 3

Breakfast: Creamy Pureed Spinach and Cheese Casserole

Lunch: Minced Tofu Stir-Fry with Soft Vegetables

Dinner: Soft-Cooked Scrambled Eggs with Cheese

DAY 4

Breakfast: Smooth Pureed Lentil Curry

Lunch: Creamy Polenta with Minced Sausage and Mushrooms

Dinner: Salmon Patties with Mashed Potatoes

DAY 5

Breakfast: Smooth Pureed Cauliflower and Cheese

Lunch: Minced Ham and Cheese Quiche

Dinner: Beef Stew with Soft Vegetables

DAY 6

Breakfast: Velvety Pureed Spinach and Potato Soup

Lunch: Minced Beef and Barley Soup

Dinner: Chicken and Vegetable Stir-Fry

DAY 7

Breakfast: Creamy Pureed Broccoli and Cheddar Bake

Lunch: Minced Chicken and Vegetable Stew

Dinner: Soft Apple Crumble with Oat Topping

DAY 8

Breakfast: Creamy Pureed Mushroom Risotto

Lunch: Creamy Mashed Potatoes with Minced Beef

Dinner: Banana Pancakes with Yogurt Topping

DAY 9

Breakfast: Rich Pureed Beef and Barley Soup

Lunch: Minced Salmon Cakes with Soft Peas

Dinner: Soft-Cooked Carrots with Honey Glaze

DAY 10

Breakfast: Pureed Chicken and Rice Congee

Lunch: Beef and Vegetable Meatloaf with Gravy

Dinner: Soft Tuna Salad with Avocado

DAY 11

Breakfast: Soft Pureed Vegetable Lasagna

Lunch: Creamy Cauliflower and Cheese Soup with Minced Chicken

Dinner: Soft-Cooked Pasta with Tomato Sauce

DAY 12

Breakfast: Pureed Chicken and Vegetable Soup

Lunch: Minced Shrimp Risotto

Dinner: Creamy Chicken and Rice Casserole

DAY 13

Breakfast: Creamy Pureed Spinach and Cheese Casserole

Lunch: Minced Tofu Stir-Fry with Soft Vegetables

Dinner: Soft-Cooked Scrambled Eggs with Cheese

DAY 14

Breakfast: Smooth Pureed Lentil Curry

Lunch: Creamy Polenta with Minced Sausage and Mushrooms

Dinner: Salmon Patties with Mashed Potatoes

CHAPTER 3

NUTRITIOUS RECIPES FOR SENIORS WITH DYSPHAGIA

LEVEL 4 PUREED

Pureed Chicken and Vegetable Soup

Preparation Time: 30 minutes

Serves:2

Calories: 320mg **Carbs:** 30g **Protein:** 30g **Fat:** 8g **Fiber:** 6g **Sodium:** 150mg

Ingredients:

1 lb. boneless, skinless chicken breast (or thigh), well cooked and shredded

2 cups carrots, peeled and chopped

2 cups celery, chopped

2 cups potatoes, peeled and diced

1 onion, chopped

4 cups low-sodium chicken broth

1 cup low-fat milk

A pinch of salt and pepper

Method of Preparation:

1. In a large pot, combine the shredded chicken, carrots, celery, potatoes, onion, and chicken broth.
2. Bring the mixture to a boil, then reduce the heat and simmer for 20-25 minutes, or until the vegetables are tender.
3. Allow the soup to cool slightly, then transfer it to a blender or food processor and puree until smooth.
4. Return the pureed soup to the pot and stir in the milk. Heat gently until warmed through.
5. Season with a salt and pepper before serving.

Creamy Pureed Spinach and Cheese Casserole

Preparation Time: 40 minutes

Serves:2

Calories: 250mg **Carbs:** 15g **Protein:** 20g **Fat:** 12g **Fiber:** 6g **Sodium:** 200mg

Ingredients:

1 lb. frozen chopped spinach, thawed and drained

1 cup low-fat cottage cheese

1/2 cup grated Parmesan cheese

2 eggs

1/4 cup low-fat milk

A pinch of salt and pepper

Pinch of nutmeg (optional)

Method of Preparation:

1. Preheat the oven to 350°F (175°C). Lightly grease a baking dish.
2. In a large bowl, combine the thawed spinach, cottage cheese, Parmesan cheese, eggs, milk, salt, pepper, and nutmeg (if using).
3. Mix well until all ingredients are thoroughly combined.

4. Transfer the mixture to the prepared baking dish and spread it out evenly.

5. Bake in the preheated oven for 25-30 minutes, or until the casserole is set and lightly golden on top.

6. Allow the casserole to cool slightly before serving.

Smooth Pureed Lentil Curry

Serves: 2

Preparation Time: 35 minutes

Calories: 280mg **Carbs:** 40g **Protein:** 20g **Fat:** 4g **Fiber:** 12g **Sodium:** 200mg

Ingredients:

1 cup dried red lentils

2 cups low-sodium vegetable broth

1 onion, chopped

2 cloves garlic, minced

1-inch piece of ginger, grated

1 tablespoon curry powder

1 teaspoon ground cumin

1 teaspoon ground coriander

1/2 teaspoon turmeric

1/4 teaspoon cayenne pepper (optional)

A pinch of salt

1 tablespoon olive oil

Method of Preparation:

1. Rinse the lentils under cold water and drain.
2. In a large pot, heat the olive oil over medium heat. Add the chopped onion, garlic, and ginger, and sauté until softened, about 5 minutes.
3. Add the curry powder, cumin, coriander, turmeric, and cayenne pepper (if using) to the pot, and cook for another minute, stirring constantly.
4. Add the lentils and vegetable broth to the pot, and bring to a boil. Reduce the heat to low, cover, and simmer for 20-25 minutes, or until the lentils are tender.
5. Allow the mixture to cool slightly, then transfer it to a blender or food processor and puree until smooth.
6. Season with salt before serving.

Smooth Pureed Cauliflower and Cheese

Preparation Time: 20 minutes

Serves:2

Calories: 180mg **Carbs:** 20g **Protein:** 20g **Fat:** 5g **Fiber:** 6g **Sodium:** 150mg

Ingredients:

1 head cauliflower, chopped into florets

1 cup low-sodium vegetable broth

1/2 cup low-fat milk

1/2 cup shredded low-fat cheddar cheese

A pinch of salt and pepper

Pinch of garlic powder (optional)

Method of Preparation:

1. Steam or boil the cauliflower florets until tender, for about 10-12 minutes.

2. In a blender or food processor, combine the cooked cauliflower, vegetable broth, milk, shredded cheddar cheese, salt, pepper, and garlic powder (if using).

3. Blend until smooth and creamy, adding more broth or milk if needed to reach desired consistency.

4. Transfer the pureed mixture to a saucepan and heat gently over low heat until warmed through.

5. Adjust seasoning with salt and pepper, if necessary, before serving.

Velvety Pureed Spinach and Potato Soup

Preparation Time: 30 minutes

Serves:2

Calories: 220mg **Carbs:** 30g **Protein:** 15g **Fat:** 4g **Fiber:** 8g **Sodium:** 250mg

Ingredients:

2 cups fresh spinach leaves

2 medium potatoes, peeled and diced

1 onion, chopped

2 cloves garlic, minced

4 cups low-sodium vegetable broth

1/2 cup low-fat milk

A pinch of salt and pepper

Pinch of nutmeg (optional)

Method of Preparation:

1. In a large pot, combine the spinach, potatoes, onion, garlic, and vegetable broth.
2. Bring the mixture to a boil, then reduce the heat and simmer for 15-20 minutes, or until the potatoes are fork-tender.
3. Allow the soup to cool slightly, then transfer it to a blender or food processor and puree until smooth.
4. Return the pureed soup to the pot and stir in the milk. Heat gently until warmed through.
5. Season with salt, pepper, and nutmeg (if using) before serving.

Creamy Pureed Broccoli and Cheddar Bake

Preparation Time: 40 minutes

Serves: 2

Calories: 250mg **Carbs:** 25g **Protein:** 15g **Fat:** 8g

 Fiber: 8g **Sodium:** 450mg

Ingredients:

1 lb. broccoli florets

1 cup low-sodium vegetable broth

1/2 cup low-fat milk

1/2 cup shredded low-fat cheddar cheese

2 tablespoons whole wheat flour

1 tablespoon olive oil

A pinch of salt

Pinch of paprika (optional)

Method of Preparation:

1. Steam or boil the broccoli florets until tender, about 8-10 minutes.

2. Drain well.

3. In a saucepan, heat the olive oil over medium heat. Stir in the whole wheat flour and cook for 1-2 minutes, until lightly golden.

4. Gradually whisk in the vegetable broth and milk, stirring constantly until the mixture thickens.

5. Remove the saucepan from the heat and stir in the shredded cheddar cheese until melted and smooth.

6. In a large bowl, combine the cooked broccoli with the cheese sauce, and mix well to coat.

7. Transfer the mixture to a baking dish and sprinkle with a pinch of paprika (if using).

8. Bake in a preheated oven at 375°F (190°C) for 20-25 minutes, or until bubbly and golden on top.

9. Allow the bake to cool slightly before serving.

Creamy Pureed Mushroom Risotto

Preparation Time: 40 minutes

Serves: 2

Calories: 350mg **Carbs:** 50g **Protein:** 18g **Fat:** 12g **Fiber:** 4g **Sodium:** 500mg

Ingredients:

1 cup Arborio rice

2 cups low-sodium vegetable broth

1 cup mushrooms, sliced

1/2 onion, finely chopped

2 cloves garlic, minced

1/4 cup grated Parmesan cheese

1/4 cup low-fat milk

2 tablespoons olive oil

A pinch of salt

Method of Preparation:

1. In a large saucepan, heat the olive oil over medium heat.

2. Add the chopped onion and minced garlic, and sauté until softened, about 3-4 minutes.

3. Add the sliced mushrooms to the saucepan and cook until they release their juices and become tender, about 5-6 minutes.

4. Stir in the Arborio rice and cook for another 2-3 minutes, until lightly toasted.

5. Gradually add the vegetable broth to the saucepan, one ladleful at a time, stirring frequently and allowing the liquid to be absorbed before adding more.

6. Continue cooking and stirring until the rice is creamy and tender, about 20-25 minutes.

7. Stir in the grated Parmesan cheese and low-fat milk, and season with salt.

8. Allow the risotto to cool slightly, then transfer it to a blender or food processor and puree until smooth.

9. Serve the creamy pureed mushroom risotto warm, garnished with additional grated Parmesan cheese if desired.

Rich Pureed Beef and Barley Soup

Preparation Time: 90 minutes

Serves:2

Calories: 300mg **Carbs:** 35g **Protein:** 20g **Fat:** 8g **Fiber:** 7g **Sodium:** 300mg

Ingredients:

1/2 lb. lean beef stew meat, diced

1/2 cup pearl barley

2 carrots, peeled and chopped

2 celery stalks, chopped

1 onion, chopped

2 cloves garlic, minced

4 cups low-sodium beef broth

A pinch of salt and pepper

Method of Preparation:

1. In a large pot, combine the diced beef stew meat, pearl barley, chopped carrots, celery, onion, garlic, and beef broth.
2. Bring the mixture to a boil, then reduce the heat and simmer for 1-1.5 hours, or until the beef is tender and the barley is cooked through.

3. Allow the soup to cool slightly, then transfer it to a blender or food processor and puree until smooth.

4. Return the pureed soup to the pot and heat gently until warmed through.

5. Season with salt and pepper before serving.

Pureed Chicken and Rice Congee

Preparation Time: 60 minutes

Serves:2

Calories: 250mg **Carbs:** 30g **Protein:** 20g **Fat:** 5g **Fiber:** 1g **Sodium:** 200mg

Ingredients:

1/2 cup white rice

2 cups low-sodium chicken broth

1 boneless, skinless chicken breast, cooked and shredded

1/2-inch piece of ginger, grated

2 cloves garlic, minced

A pinch of salt and pepper

Method of Preparation:

1. In a large pot, combine the white rice, low-sodium chicken broth, shredded chicken breast, grated ginger, and minced garlic.
2. Bring the mixture to a boil, then reduce the heat and simmer for 45-60 minutes, or until the rice is soft and the congee is thick and creamy.
3. Allow the congee to cool slightly, then transfer it to a blender or food processor and puree until smooth.
4. Return the pureed congee to the pot and heat gently until warmed through.
5. Season with salt and pepper before serving.

Soft Pureed Vegetable Lasagna

Preparation Time: 60 minutes

Serves: 2

Calories: 350mg **Carbs:** 45g **Protein:** 20g **Fat:** 10g **Fiber:** 5g **Sodium:** 210mg

Ingredients:

6 lasagna noodles

2 cups mixed vegetables (such as zucchini, bell peppers, mushrooms), chopped

1 cup low-fat ricotta cheese

1/2 cup grated Parmesan cheese

1/4 cup low-fat milk

1/4 cup low-sodium vegetable broth

2 cloves garlic, minced

A pinch of salt and pepper

1 tablespoon olive oil

Method of Preparation:

1. Preheat the oven to 375°F (190°C).
2. Cook the lasagna noodles according to package instructions, then drain and set aside.
3. In a large skillet, heat the olive oil over medium heat.
4. Add the minced garlic and chopped mixed vegetables, and sauté until tender, about 5-6 minutes.
5. In a mixing bowl, combine the low-fat ricotta cheese, grated Parmesan cheese, low-fat milk, and low-sodium vegetable broth.

6. Mix well to form a creamy sauce.

7. Spread a thin layer of the creamy sauce on the bottom of a baking dish.

8. Arrange 2 cooked lasagna noodles on top.

9. Spread half of the sautéed mixed vegetables over the noodles, then top with another layer of noodles.

10. Repeat the layers with the remaining vegetables and noodles, finishing with a layer of noodles on top.

11. Spread the remaining creamy sauce evenly over the top layer of noodles.

12. Cover the baking dish with foil and bake in the preheated oven for 25-30 minutes, or until the lasagna is heated through and bubbly.

13. Allow the lasagna to cool slightly before serving.

LEVEL 5 MINCED AND MOIST

Creamy Cauliflower and Cheese Soup with Minced Chicken

Preparation Time: 30 minutes

Serves: 2

Calories: 350mg **Carbs:** 20g **Protein:** 30g **Fat:** 15g **Fiber:** 5g **Sodium:** 300mg

Ingredients:

1 medium head cauliflower, chopped into florets

1 cup low-sodium chicken broth

1/2 lb. minced chicken breast

1/2 onion, chopped

2 cloves garlic, minced

1 cup low-fat milk

1/2 cup shredded low-fat cheddar cheese

A pinch of salt and pepper

1 tablespoon olive oil

Method of Preparation:

1. In a large pot, heat the olive oil over medium heat. Add the minced chicken, chopped onion, and minced garlic.
2. Cook until the chicken is fully cooked and the vegetables are tender, about 5-6 minutes.

3. Add the cauliflower florets to the pot, along with the chicken broth.

4. Bring to a boil, then reduce the heat and simmer until the cauliflower is soft, about 10-12 minutes.

5. Using an immersion blender or transferring to a blender in batches, puree the soup until smooth.

6. Return the soup to the pot and stir in the low-fat milk and shredded cheddar cheese until the cheese is melted and the soup is creamy.

7. Season with salt and pepper before serving.

Minced Shrimp Risotto

Preparation Time: 40 minutes

Serves:2

Calories: 380mg **Carbs:** 45g **Protein:** 25g **Fat:** 12g **Fiber:** 3g **Sodium:** 200mg

Ingredients:

1 cup Arborio rice

4 cups low-sodium vegetable broth

1/2 lb. minced shrimp

1/2 onion, finely chopped

2 cloves garlic, minced

1/4 cup grated Parmesan cheese

2 tablespoons low-fat milk

A pinch of salt and pepper

1 tablespoon olive oil

Method of Preparation:

1. In a large saucepan, heat the olive oil over medium heat.

2. Add the minced shrimp, chopped onion, and minced garlic.

3. Cook until the shrimp is pink and cooked through, about 3-4 minutes.

4. Stir in the Arborio rice and cook for another 2-3 minutes, until lightly toasted.

5. Gradually add the vegetable broth to the saucepan, one ladleful at a time, stirring frequently and allowing the liquid to be absorbed before adding more.

6. Continue cooking and stirring until the rice is creamy and tender, about 20-25 minutes.

7. Stir in the grated Parmesan cheese and low-fat milk until well combined.

8. Serve the minced shrimp risotto warm, garnished with additional grated Parmesan cheese if desired.

9. Season with salt and pepper before serving.

Minced Tofu Stir-Fry with Soft Vegetables

Preparation Time: 20 minutes

Serves:2

Calories: 280mg **Carbs:** 15g **Protein:** 20g **Fat:** 15g**Fiber:** 5g **Sodium:** 600mg

Ingredients:

1/2 lb. minced firm tofu

2 cups mixed soft vegetables (such as bell peppers, zucchini, mushrooms), chopped

1/2 onion, thinly sliced

2 cloves garlic, minced

2 tablespoons low-sodium soy sauce

1 tablespoon sesame oil

A pinch of salt and pepper

1 tablespoon olive oil

Method of Preparation:

1. In a large skillet or wok, heat the olive oil over medium-high heat.
2. Add the minced tofu and cook until lightly browned and crispy, about 5-6 minutes.
3. Remove from the skillet and set aside.
4. In the same skillet, add the sliced onion, minced garlic, and chopped soft vegetables.
5. Stir-fry until the vegetables are tender-crisp, about 4-5 minutes.
6. Return the cooked tofu to the skillet.
7. Add the low-sodium soy sauce and sesame oil, and toss to coat everything evenly.
8. Cook for another 2-3 minutes, allowing the flavors to blend together.

9. Season with salt and pepper before serving.

Creamy Polenta with Minced Sausage and Mushrooms

Preparation Time: 30 minutes

Serves:2

Calories: 400mg **Carbs:** 20g **Protein:** 20g **Fat:** 9g **Fiber:** 4g **Sodium:** 300mg

Ingredients:

1 cup yellow cornmeal (polenta)

4 cups low-sodium chicken or vegetable broth

1/2 lb. minced sausage (choose a low-fat option)

1 cup mushrooms, sliced

1/2 onion, finely chopped

2 cloves garlic, minced

1/4 cup grated Parmesan cheese

2 tablespoons low-fat milk

A pinch of salt and pepper

Method of Preparation:

1. In a large saucepan, bring the chicken or vegetable broth to a boil.

2. Gradually whisk in the yellow cornmeal, stirring constantly to prevent lumps from forming.

3. Reduce the heat to low and simmer, stirring occasionally, for 20-25 minutes or until the polenta is thick and creamy.

4. While the polenta cooks, heat a skillet over medium heat. Add the minced sausage, mushrooms, onion, and garlic. Cook until the sausage is browned and the vegetables are tender, about 8-10 minutes.

5. Once the polenta is cooked, stir in the grated Parmesan cheese and low-fat milk until well combined.

6. Serve the creamy polenta topped with the cooked sausage and mushroom mixture.

7. Season with salt and pepper before serving.

Minced Ham and Cheese Quiche

Preparation Time: 40 minutes

Serves:2

Calories: 350mg **Carbs:** 10g **Protein:** 25g **Fat:** 9g **Fiber:** 4g **Sodium:** 200mg

Ingredients:

1 pre-made pie crust (choose a low-fat option, if available)

1 cup minced ham

1/2 cup low-fat shredded cheddar cheese

4 eggs

1/2 cup low-fat milk

A pinch of salt and pepper

Method of Preparation:

1. Preheat the oven to 375°F (190°C).
2. Place the pre-made pie crust in a pie dish and crimp the edges.
3. In a mixing bowl, combine the minced ham and shredded cheddar cheese.
4. Spread the mixture evenly over the bottom of the pie crust.
5. In another mixing bowl, whisk together the eggs and low-fat milk.

6. Season with salt and pepper.

7. Pour the egg mixture over the ham and cheese in the pie crust.

8. Bake in the preheated oven for 30-35 minutes, or until the quiche is set and the crust is golden brown.

9. Allow the quiche to cool slightly before slicing and serving.

Minced Beef and Barley Soup

Preparation Time: 60 minutes

Serves:2

Calories: 300mg **Carbs:** 15g **Protein:** 25g **Fat:** 5g **Fiber:** 6g **Sodium:** 200mg

Ingredients:

1/2 lb. lean minced beef

1/2 cup pearl barley

2 carrots, peeled and chopped

2 celery stalks, chopped

1 onion, chopped

2 cloves garlic, minced

4 cups low-sodium beef broth

A pinch of salt and pepper

Method of Preparation:

1. In a large pot, brown the minced beef over medium heat until fully cooked, breaking it up with a spoon as it cooks.
2. Add the chopped carrots, celery, onion, and minced garlic to the pot.
3. Cook for another 5-6 minutes, until the vegetables are tender.
4. Stir in the pearl barley and beef broth.
5. Bring the mixture to a boil, then reduce the heat and simmer for 45-60 minutes, or until the barley is tender.
6. Season the soup with salt and pepper before serving.

Minced Chicken and Vegetable Stew

Preparation Time: 30 minutes

Serves: 2

Calories: 280mg **Carbs:** 15g **Protein:** 20g **Fat:** 12g **Fiber:** 3g **Sodium:** 200mg

Ingredients:

1/2 lb. minced chicken breast

2 carrots, peeled and chopped

2 celery stalks, chopped

1 onion, chopped

2 cloves garlic, minced

2 cups low-sodium chicken broth

1 tablespoon tomato paste

1 teaspoon dried thyme

A pinch of salt and pepper

1 tablespoon olive oil

Method of Preparation:

1. In a large pot, heat the olive oil over medium heat.
2. Add the minced chicken, chopped carrots, celery, onion, and minced garlic.

3. Cook until the chicken is fully cooked and the vegetables are tender, about 5-6 minutes.

4. Stir in the tomato paste and dried thyme, and cook for another minute.

5. Add the low-sodium chicken broth to the pot, and bring to a boil.

6. Reduce the heat and simmer for 20-25 minutes, allowing the flavors to meld together.

7. Season with salt and pepper before serving.

Creamy Mashed Potatoes with Minced Beef

Preparation Time: 30 minutes

Serves:2

Calories: 320mg **Carbs:** 25g **Protein:** 20g **Fat:** 15g **Fiber:** 4g **Sodium:** 250mg

Ingredients:

2 medium potatoes, peeled and diced

1/2 lb. minced beef

1/2 onion, chopped

1 clove garlic, minced

1/4 cup low-fat milk

A pinch of salt and pepper

1 tablespoon olive oil

Method of Preparation:

1. Place the diced potatoes in a pot of water and bring
   to a boil.
2. Cook until the potatoes are fork-tender, about 15-20
   minutes.
3. Drain well.
4. In a large skillet, heat the olive oil over medium heat.
5. Add the minced beef, chopped onion, and minced
   garlic.
6. Cook until the beef is browned and cooked through,
   breaking it up with a spoon as it cooks.
7. Mash the cooked potatoes with a potato masher or
   fork until smooth.
8. Stir in the low-fat milk until creamy.
9. Serve the creamy mashed potatoes topped with the
   cooked minced beef mixture.

10. Season with A pinch of salt and pepper before serving.

Minced Salmon Cakes with Soft Peas

Preparation Time: 20 minutes

Serves: 2

Calories: 300mg **Carbs:** 20g **Protein:** 25g **Fat:** 15g **Fiber:** 5g **Sodium:** 200mg

Ingredients:

1/2 lb. minced salmon

1/4 cup breadcrumbs (choose a soft variety)

1 egg

2 tablespoons chopped fresh dill

1/4 teaspoon garlic powder

A pinch of A pinch of salt and pepper

1 tablespoon olive oil

1 cup frozen peas, thawed

Method of Preparation:

1. In a mixing bowl, combine the minced salmon, breadcrumbs, egg, chopped fresh dill, garlic powder, salt, and pepper.
2. Mix until well combined.
3. Divide the mixture into equal portions and shape into patties.
4. Heat the olive oil in a skillet over medium heat.
5. Add the salmon patties and cook until golden brown and cooked through, about 3-4 minutes per side.
6. Serve the minced salmon cakes with the thawed peas on the side.

Beef and Vegetable Meatloaf with Gravy

Preparation Time: 60 minutes

Serves:2

Calories: 135mg **Carbs:** 10g **Protein:** 25g **Fat:** 8g **Fiber:** 3g **Sodium:** 200mg

Ingredients:

1/2 lb. minced beef

1/2 onion, chopped

1 carrot, peeled and grated

1 celery stalk, chopped

1/4 cup breadcrumbs (choose a soft variety)

1 egg

1 tablespoon Worcestershire sauce

A pinch of salt and pepper

1 cup low-sodium beef broth

1 tablespoon cornstarch

1 tablespoon water

Method of Preparation:

1. Preheat the oven to 375°F (190°C).
2. Lightly grease a loaf pan.

3. In a mixing bowl, combine the minced beef, chopped onion, grated carrot, chopped celery, breadcrumbs, egg, Worcestershire sauce, salt, and pepper.

4. Mix until well combined.

5. Press the mixture into the prepared loaf pan, smoothing the top with a spoon.

6. Bake in the preheated oven for 45-50 minutes, or until the meatloaf is cooked through and golden brown on top.

7. In a small saucepan, combine the low-sodium beef broth, cornstarch, and water.

8. Cook over medium heat, stirring constantly, until the gravy thickens.

9. Serve slices of the beef and vegetable meatloaf with the gravy on top.

LEVEL 6 SOFT AND BITE-SIZED

Soft-Cooked Carrots with Honey Glaze

Preparation Time: 15 minutes

Serves:2

Calories: 50mg **Carbs:** 8g **Protein:** 10g **Fat:** 5g **Fiber:** 3g **Sodium:** 50mg

Ingredients:

2 large carrots, peeled and sliced into coins

1 tablespoon honey

1 cup chicken broth

1 tablespoon unsalted butter

A pinch of salt

Method of Preparation:

1. Boil the carrot slices until they are tender in the chicken broth about 5-7 minutes.
2. In a small saucepan, melt the unsalted butter over low heat.
3. Add the honey and a pinch of salt to the melted butter, stirring until combined.
4. Pour the honey glaze over the cooked carrots and toss gently to coat.
5. Serve the soft-cooked carrots with honey glaze warm.

Banana Pancakes with Yogurt Topping

Preparation Time: 15 minutes

Serves:2

Calories: 100mg **Carbs:** 15g **Protein:** 8g **Fat:** 5g **Fiber:** 5g **Sodium:** 50mg

Ingredients:

1 ripe banana

1 egg

1/4 cup oat flour (or finely ground oats)

1/4 teaspoon baking powder

1/4 teaspoon cinnamon (optional)

1/4 cup low-fat yogurt

1 tablespoon honey (optional)

Method of Preparation:

1. In a mixing bowl, mash the ripe banana until smooth.

2. Add the egg, oat flour, baking powder, and cinnamon (if using) to the mashed banana.

3. Mix until well combined.

4. Heat a non-stick skillet over medium heat.

5. Pour small portions of the pancake batter onto the skillet, using about 2 tablespoons of batter per pancake.

6. Cook the pancakes for 2-3 minutes on each side, or until golden brown and cooked through.

7. Serve the banana pancakes topped with low-fat yogurt and drizzled with honey (if desired).

Soft Apple Crumble with Oat Topping

Preparation Time: 35 minutes

Serves:2

Calories: 100mg **Carbs:** 23g **Protein:** 10g **Fat:** 7g **Fiber:** 5g **Sodium:** 25mg

Ingredients:

2 medium apples, peeled, cored, and sliced

1 tablespoon lemon juice

1/4 teaspoon cinnamon

1/4 cup rolled oats

1 tablespoon unsalted butter, melted

1 tablespoon honey

A pinch of salt

Method of Preparation:

1. Preheat the oven to 350°F (175°C).
2. Lightly grease a small baking dish.
3. In a mixing bowl, toss the sliced apples with lemon juice and cinnamon until evenly coated.
4. Spread the apple slices in the prepared baking dish.
5. In the same mixing bowl, combine the rolled oats, melted unsalted butter, honey, and a pinch of salt.
6. Mix until crumbly.
7. Sprinkle the oat topping evenly over the apple slices.
8. Bake in the preheated oven for 25-30 minutes, or until the apples are soft and the topping is golden brown.
9. Serve the soft apple crumble warm.

Chicken and Vegetable Stir-Fry

Preparation Time: 20 minutes

Serves:2

Calories: 150mg **Carbs:** 8g **Protein:** 25g **Fat:** 5g **Fiber:** 4g
Sodium: 250mg

Ingredients:

1/2 lb. boneless, skinless chicken breast, thinly sliced

1 cup mixed vegetables (such as bell peppers, broccoli, carrots), sliced

1/2 onion, sliced

2 cloves garlic, minced

2 tablespoons low-sodium soy sauce

1 tablespoon olive oil

A pinch of salt and pepper

Method of Preparation:

1. Heat the olive oil in a large skillet or wok over medium-high heat.

2. Add the sliced chicken breast to the skillet and cook until no longer pink, about 5-6 minutes.

3. Add the sliced mixed vegetables, sliced onion, and minced garlic to the skillet.

4. Stir-fry until the vegetables are tender-crisp, about 4-5 minutes.

5. Stir in the low-sodium soy sauce and continue to cook for another 1-2 minutes.

6. Season with salt and pepper.

7. Serve the chicken and vegetable stir-fry hot.

Beef Stew with Soft Vegetables

Preparation Time: 90 minutes

Serves:2

Calories: 125mg **Carbs:** 15g **Protein:** 25g **Fat:** 5g **Fiber:** 5g **Sodium:** 300mg

Ingredients:

1/2 lb. stewing beef, cut into bite-sized pieces

2 carrots, peeled and chopped

2 potatoes, peeled and chopped

1/2 onion, chopped

2 cloves garlic, minced

2 cups low-sodium beef broth

1 tablespoon tomato paste

1/2 teaspoon dried thyme

A pinch of salt and pepper

Method of Preparation:

1. In a large pot, heat some olive oil over medium heat.
2. Add the chopped onions and minced garlic, and cook until softened for about 3-4 minutes.
3. Add the beef to the pot and cook until browned on all sides.
4. Stir in the chopped carrots, potatoes, beef broth, tomato paste, and dried thyme.
5. Bring to a boil.
6. Reduce the heat to low, cover, and simmer for 1 to 1.5 hours, or until the beef and vegetables are tender.
7. Season with salt and pepper before serving.

Salmon Patties with Mashed Potatoes

Preparation Time: 30 minutes

Serves:2

Calories: 200mg **Carbs:** 15g **Protein:** 25g **Fat:** 15g **Fiber:** 4g **Sodium:** 200mg

Ingredients:

1/2 lb. canned salmon, drained and flaked

1/4 cup breadcrumbs (choose a soft variety)

1 egg

1 tablespoon chopped fresh parsley

1/4 teaspoon garlic powder

A pinch of salt and pepper

2 medium potatoes, peeled and diced

1/4 cup low-fat milk

1 tablespoon unsalted butter

Method of Preparation:

1. In a mixing bowl, combine the flaked salmon, breadcrumbs, egg, chopped parsley, garlic powder, salt, and pepper.
2. Mix until well combined.
3. Divide the mixture into equal portions and shape into patties.
4. Heat some olive oil in a skillet over medium heat.
5. Cook the salmon patties until golden brown on both sides, about 3-4 minutes per side.
6. Meanwhile, cook the diced potatoes in boiling water until tender, about 15 minutes.
7. Drain well.
8. Mash the cooked potatoes with low-fat milk, unsalted butter, and a pinch of salt until smooth and creamy.
9. Serve the salmon patties with mashed potatoes.

Soft-Cooked Scrambled Eggs with Cheese

Preparation Time: 10 minutes

Serves:2

Calories: 125mg **Carbs:** 3g **Protein:** 15g **Fat:** 9g **Fiber:** 2g
Sodium: 150mg

Ingredients:

4 eggs

1/4 cup low-fat milk

1/4 cup shredded low-fat cheese

A pinch of salt and pepper

1 tablespoon unsalted butter

Method of Preparation:

1. Crack the eggs into a mixing bowl and beat lightly with a fork.
2. Stir in the low-fat milk, shredded cheese, salt, and pepper.
3. Melt the unsalted butter in a non-stick skillet over low heat.
4. Pour the egg mixture into the skillet and cook gently, stirring constantly, until the eggs are softly scrambled and the cheese is melted.

5. Serve the soft-cooked scrambled eggs with cheese hot.

Creamy Chicken and Rice Casserole

Preparation Time: 30 minutes

Serves:2

Calories: 125mg **Carbs:** 15g **Protein:** 30g **Fat:** 12g **Fiber:** 2g **Sodium:** 200mg

Ingredients:

1/2 lb. boneless, skinless chicken breast, cooked and shredded

1 cup cooked white rice

1/2 cup low-fat sour cream

1/2 cup low-sodium chicken broth

1/4 cup shredded low-fat cheese

1/4 cup frozen peas, thawed

A pinch of salt and pepper

Method of Preparation:

1. Preheat the oven to 375°F (190°C).
2. Lightly grease a small baking dish.
3. In a mixing bowl, combine the shredded chicken, cooked white rice, low-fat sour cream, low-sodium chicken broth, shredded cheese, thawed peas, salt, and pepper.
4. Transfer the mixture to the prepared baking dish and spread it out evenly.
5. Bake in the preheated oven for 20-25 minutes, or until heated through and bubbly.
6. Serve the creamy chicken and rice casserole hot.

Soft-Cooked Pasta with Tomato Sauce

Preparation Time: 15 minutes

Serves: 2

Calories: 100mg **Carbs:** 15g **Protein:** 8g **Fat:** 2g **Fiber:** 4g
Sodium: 150mg

Ingredients:

1 cup cooked pasta (choose a soft variety)

1/2 cup tomato sauce

1 tablespoon grated Parmesan cheese

Fresh basil leaves for garnish (optional)

Method of Preparation:

1. Cook the pasta according to package instructions until al dente.
2. Drain well.
3. In a small saucepan, heat the tomato sauce over low heat until warmed through.
4. Pour the warm tomato sauce over the cooked pasta and toss to coat evenly.
5. Sprinkle grated Parmesan cheese over the pasta.
6. Garnish with fresh basil leaves, if desired.
7. Serve the soft-cooked pasta with tomato sauce hot.

Soft Tuna Salad with Avocado

Preparation Time: 10 minutes

Serves: 2

Calories: 125mg **Carbs:** 5g **Protein:** 20g **Fat:** 8g **Fiber:** 7g **Sodium:** 150mg

Ingredients:

1 can (5 oz) tuna in water, drained

1 ripe avocado, mashed

2 tablespoons low-fat mayonnaise

1 tablespoon lemon juice

A pinch of salt and pepper

Whole grain bread for serving (optional)

Method of Preparation:

1. In a mixing bowl, combine the drained tuna, mashed avocado, low-fat mayonnaise, lemon juice, salt, and pepper.
2. Mix until well combined.
3. Serve the soft tuna salad with whole grain bread if desired.

Berry Yogurt Parfait

Preparation Time: 5 minutes

Serves:2

Calories: 100mg **Carbs:** 15g **Protein:** 8g **Fat:** 5g **Fiber:** 4g **Sodium:** 100mg

Ingredients:

1 cup low-fat yogurt

1/2 cup mixed berries (such as strawberries, blueberries, raspberries)

1/4 cup granola

1 tablespoon honey (optional)

Method of Preparation:

1. In a serving glass or bowl, layer the low-fat yogurt, mixed berries, and granola.
2. Drizzle honey over the top, if desired.
3. Repeat the layers until the glass or bowl is filled.
4. Serve the berry yogurt parfait immediately.

Coconut Milk Custard

Preparation Time: 60 minutes

Serves: 2

Calories: 150mg **Carbs:** 10g **Protein:** 8g **Fat:** 25g **Fiber:** 2g **Sodium:** 50mg

Ingredients:

1 can (13.5 oz) coconut milk

3 eggs

1/4 cup honey or maple syrup

1 teaspoon vanilla extract

A pinch of salt

Fresh berries for garnish (optional)

Method of Preparation:

1. Preheat the oven to 325°F (160°C).
2. Grease two ramekins or small baking dishes.
3. In a mixing bowl, whisk together the coconut milk, eggs, honey or maple syrup, vanilla extract, and a pinch of salt until well combined.

4. Pour the custard mixture into the prepared ramekins.

5. Place the ramekins in a baking dish and fill the dish with enough hot water to reach halfway up the sides of the ramekins.

6. Bake in the preheated oven for 30-35 minutes, or until the custard is set but still slightly jiggly in the center.

7. Remove the custard from the oven and let it cool to room temperature.

8. Refrigerate for at least 1 hour before serving.

9. Garnish with fresh berries, if desired, before serving.

Avocado Chocolate Mousse

Preparation Time: 10 minutes

Serves:2

Calories: 50mg **Carbs:** 5g **Protein:** 7g **Fat:** 4g **Fiber:** 7g **Sodium:** 25mg

Ingredients:

1 ripe avocado

2 tablespoons unsweetened cocoa powder

2 tablespoons honey or maple syrup

1/4 cup low-fat milk or almond milk

1/2 teaspoon vanilla extract

A pinch of salt

Fresh berries for garnish (optional)

Method of Preparation:

1. Scoop the flesh of the ripe avocado into a blender or food processor.
2. Add the unsweetened cocoa powder, honey or maple syrup, low-fat milk or almond milk, vanilla extract, and a pinch of salt.
3. Blend until smooth and creamy, scraping down the sides of the blender or food processor as needed.
4. Divide the avocado chocolate mousse into serving glasses or bowls.
5. Refrigerate for at least 30 minutes before serving.
6. Garnish with fresh berries, if desired, before serving.

Pumpkin Pie Smoothie

Preparation Time: 5 minutes

Serves:2

Calories: 100mg **Carbs:** 20g **Protein:** 7g **Fat:** 2g **Fiber:** 6g **Sodium:** 25mg

Ingredients:

1/2 cup canned pumpkin puree

1 ripe banana

1/2 cup low-fat yogurt or almond milk

1/4 cup rolled oats

1 tablespoon honey or maple syrup

1/2 teaspoon pumpkin pie spice

Whipped cream for garnish (optional)

Method of Preparation:

1. In a blender, combine the canned pumpkin puree, ripe banana, low-fat yogurt or almond milk, rolled oats, honey or maple syrup, and pumpkin pie spice.
2. Blend until smooth and creamy.
3. Pour the pumpkin pie smoothie into serving glasses.

4. Garnish with whipped cream and a sprinkle of pumpkin pie spice, if desired, before serving.

Banana Pudding

Preparation Time: 15 minutes (plus chilling time)

Serves:2

Calories: 100mg **Carbs:** 20g **Protein:** 5g **Fat:** 2g **Fiber:** 4g

Sodium: 25mg

Ingredients:

2 ripe bananas

1/2 cup low-fat milk or almond milk

1 tablespoon cornstarch

1 tablespoon honey or maple syrup

1/2 teaspoon vanilla extract

A pinch of salt

Low-fat vanilla wafers for serving (optional)

Method of Preparation:

1. In a blender or food processor, combine the ripe bananas, low-fat milk or almond milk, cornstarch, honey or maple syrup, vanilla extract, and a pinch of salt.

2. Blend until smooth and creamy.

3. Transfer the mixture to a saucepan and cook over medium heat, stirring constantly, until thickened.

4. Remove from heat and let the banana pudding cool to room temperature.

5. Refrigerate for at least 1 hour before serving.

SMOOTHIE

Berry Blend Smoothie

Preparation Time: 5 minutes

Serves:2

Calories: 80mg **Carbs:** 15g **Protein:** 6g **Fat:** 1g **Fiber:** 5g
Sodium: 25mg

Ingredients:

1 cup mixed berries (such as strawberries, blueberries, raspberries)

1 ripe banana

1/2 cup low-fat yogurt or almond milk

1 tablespoon honey or maple syrup

Method of Preparation:

1. In a blender, combine the mixed berries, ripe banana, low-fat yogurt or almond milk, and honey or maple syrup.
2. Blend until smooth and creamy.
3. Pour the berry blend smoothie into serving glasses.
4. Serve immediately.

Peach and Mango Smoothie

Preparation Time: 5 minutes

Serves:2

Calories: 80mg **Carbs:** 17g **Protein:** 7g **Fat:** 1g **Fiber:** 4g **Sodium:** 25mg

Ingredients:

1 ripe peach, pitted and chopped

1/2 ripe mango, peeled and chopped

1/2 cup low-fat yogurt or almond milk

1 tablespoon honey or maple syrup

Method of Preparation:

1. In a blender, combine the chopped peach, chopped mango, low-fat yogurt or almond milk, and honey or maple syrup.
2. Blend until smooth and creamy.
3. Pour the peach and mango smoothie into serving glasses.
4. Serve immediately.

Avocado and Spinach Smoothie

Preparation Time: 5 minutes

Serves: 2

Calories: 100mg **Carbs:** 18g **Protein:** 7g **Fat:** 5g **Fiber:** 7g

Sodium: 50mg

Ingredients:

1 ripe avocado

1 cup fresh spinach leaves

1 ripe banana

1/2 cup low-fat yogurt or almond milk

1 tablespoon honey or maple syrup

Method of Preparation:

1. In a blender, combine the ripe avocado, fresh spinach leaves, ripe banana, low-fat yogurt or almond milk, and honey or maple syrup.
2. Blend until smooth and creamy.
3. Pour the avocado and spinach smoothie into serving glasses.
4. Serve immediately.

Apple and Cinnamon Smoothie

Preparation Time: 5 minutes

Serves: 2

Calories: 90mg **Carbs:** 19g **Protein:** 4g **Fat:** 1g **Fiber:** 5g **Sodium:** 25mg

Ingredients:

1 apple, cored and chopped

1 ripe banana

1/2 teaspoon ground cinnamon

1/2 cup low-fat yogurt or almond milk

1 tablespoon honey or maple syrup

Method of Preparation:

1. In a blender, combine the chopped apple, ripe banana, ground cinnamon, low-fat yogurt or almond milk, and honey or maple syrup.
2. Blend until smooth and creamy.
3. Pour the apple and cinnamon smoothie into serving glasses.
4. Serve immediately.

Kiwi and Strawberry Smoothie

Preparation Time: 5 minutes

Serves:2

Calories: 80mg **Carbs:** 19g **Protein:** 5g **Fat:** 1g**Fiber:** 7g **Sodium:** 25mg

Ingredients:

2 kiwis, peeled and chopped

1 cup fresh strawberries, hulled and chopped

1 ripe banana

1/2 cup low-fat yogurt or almond milk

1 tablespoon honey or maple syrup

Method of Preparation:

1. In a blender, combine the chopped kiwis, chopped strawberries, ripe banana, low-fat yogurt or almond milk, and honey or maple syrup.
2. Blend until smooth and creamy.
3. Pour the kiwi and strawberry smoothie into serving glasses.
4. Serve immediately.

Pureed Lentil Soup

Preparation Time: 40 minutes

Serves:2

Calories: 125mg **Carbs:** 20g **Protein:** 15g **Fat:** 4g **Fiber:** 15g **Sodium:** 250mg

Ingredients:

1 cup dried lentils, rinsed and drained

4 cups low-sodium vegetable broth

1 onion, chopped

2 carrots, peeled and chopped

2 celery stalks, chopped

2 cloves garlic, minced

1 teaspoon ground cumin

1/2 teaspoon ground coriander

A pinch of salt and pepper

1 tablespoon olive oil

Method of Preparation:

1. In a large pot, heat the olive oil over medium heat.
2. Add the chopped onion, carrots, celery, and minced garlic.
3. Cook until the vegetables are softened, about 5-6 minutes.
4. Add the rinsed lentils, vegetable broth, ground cumin, ground coriander, salt, and pepper to the pot.
5. Bring to a boil.
6. Reduce the heat to low, cover, and simmer for 20-25 minutes, or until the lentils are tender.
7. Use an immersion blender to puree the soup until smooth.
8. Alternatively, carefully transfer the soup in batches to a blender and blend until smooth.
9. Adjust the seasoning with salt and pepper if needed.
10. Serve the pureed lentil soup hot.

Butternut Squash Soup

Preparation Time: 45 minutes

Serves:2

Calories: 100mg **Carbs:** 23g **Protein:** 8g **Fat:** 3g **Fiber:** 10g **Sodium:** 200mg

Ingredients:

1 small butternut squash, peeled, seeded, and chopped

1 onion, chopped

2 carrots, peeled and chopped

2 celery stalks, chopped

2 cloves garlic, minced

4 cups low-sodium vegetable broth

1/2 teaspoon ground cinnamon

1/4 teaspoon ground nutmeg

A pinch of salt and pepper

1 tablespoon olive oil

Method of Preparation:

1. In a large pot, heat the olive oil over medium heat.

2. Add the chopped onion, carrots, celery, and minced garlic.

3. Cook until the vegetables are softened, about 5-6 minutes.

4. Add the chopped butternut squash, vegetable broth, ground cinnamon, ground nutmeg, salt, and pepper to the pot.

5. Bring to a boil.

6. Reduce the heat to low, cover, and simmer for 20-25 minutes, or until the butternut squash is tender.

7. Use an immersion blender to puree the soup until smooth.

8. Alternatively, carefully transfer the soup in batches to a blender and blend until smooth.

9. Adjust the seasoning with salt and pepper if needed.

10. Serve the butternut squash soup hot.

Chicken and Rice Soup

Preparation Time: 40 minutes

Serves:2

Calories: 125mg **Carbs:** 15g **Protein:** 20g **Fat:** 5g **Fiber:** 4g **Sodium:** 250mg

Ingredients:

1 boneless, skinless chicken breast

4 cups low-sodium chicken broth

1/2 cup cooked white rice

1 carrot, peeled and chopped

1 celery stalk, chopped

1/2 onion, chopped

2 cloves garlic, minced

A pinch of salt and pepper

1 tablespoon olive oil

Method of Preparation:

1. In a large pot, heat the olive oil over medium heat.
2. Add the chopped onion, carrot, celery, and minced garlic.
3. Cook until the vegetables are softened, about 5-6 minutes.
4. Add the boneless, skinless chicken breast and low-sodium chicken broth to the pot.

5. Bring to a boil.

6. Reduce the heat to low, cover, and simmer for 20-25 minutes, or until the chicken is cooked through.

7. Remove the chicken breast from the pot and shred it using two forks.

8. Return the shredded chicken to the pot.

9. Stir in the cooked white rice and season with salt and.

10. Serve the chicken and rice soup hot.

Puréed Beef Stew

Preparation Time: 90 minutes

Serves:2

Calories: 150mg **Carbs:** 15g **Protein:** 25g **Fat:** 10g **Fiber:** 5g **Sodium:** 200mg

Ingredients:

1/2 lb. beef stew meat, cubed

1 onion, chopped

2 carrots, peeled and chopped

2 potatoes, peeled and chopped

2 cloves garlic, minced

4 cups low-sodium beef broth

1 tablespoon tomato paste

1/2 teaspoon dried thyme

A pinch of salt and pepper

1 tablespoon olive oil

Method of Preparation:

1. In a large pot, heat the olive oil over medium heat.
2. Add the chopped onion and minced garlic.
3. Cook until softened, about 3-4 minutes.
4. Add the cubed beef stew meat to the pot and cook until browned on all sides.
5. Stir in the chopped carrots, potatoes, low-sodium beef broth, tomato paste, dried thyme, salt, and pepper.
6. Bring the stew to a boil, then reduce the heat to low, cover, and simmer for 1 to 1.5 hours, or until the beef and vegetables are tender.
7. Allow the stew to cool slightly, then use an immersion blender to puree the stew until smooth.

Alternatively, carefully transfer the stew in batches to a blender and blend until smooth.

8. Adjust the seasoning with salt and pepper if needed.

9. Serve the puréed beef stew hot.

Chicken and Tomato Stew

Preparation Time: 40 minutes

Serves:2

Calories: 125g **Carbs:** 10g **Protein:** 25g **Fat:** 8g **Fiber:** 5g **Sodium:** 250mg

Ingredients:

1 boneless, skinless chicken breast, cubed

1 onion, chopped

2 tomatoes, chopped

1 carrot, peeled and chopped

1 celery stalk, chopped

2 cloves garlic, minced

2 cups low-sodium chicken broth

1/2 teaspoon dried basil

A pinch of salt and pepper

1 tablespoon olive oil

Method of Preparation:

1. In a large pot, heat the olive oil over medium heat. Add the chopped onion and minced garlic.
2. Cook until softened, about 3-4 minutes.
3. Add the cubed chicken breast to the pot and cook until browned on all sides.
4. Stir in the chopped tomatoes, carrot, celery, low-sodium chicken broth, dried basil, salt, and pepper.
5. Bring the stew to a boil, then reduce the heat to low, cover, and simmer for 20-25 minutes, or until the chicken is cooked through and the vegetables are tender.
6. Adjust the seasoning with salt and pepper if needed.
7. Serve the chicken and tomato stew hot.

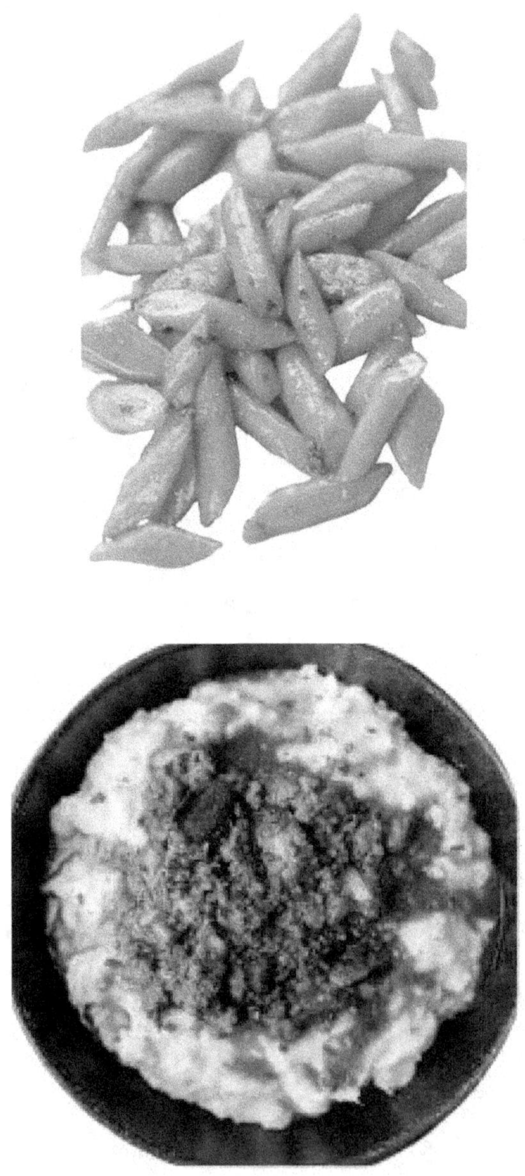

CONCLUSION

In conclusion, this book serves as a valuable resource, providing you with practical solutions and delicious recipes carefully crafted to soothe your unique dietary needs and challenges associated with dysphagia.

Through the careful selection of ingredients and meticulous attention to food texture and consistency, the dysphagia cookbook offers you a diverse array of flavorful meals that are not only safe to consume but also enjoyable and satisfying.

More so, this book goes beyond mere recipe compilation, it also serves as an educational tool to enhance seniors' understanding of dysphagia and its management.

Each recipe is accompanied by helpful tips and guidelines for safe swallowing, empowering you to make informed choices and adopt healthy eating habits that promotes optimal nutrition and overall well-being.

By equipping you with the tools and knowledge you need to navigate your dietary restrictions with confidence and creativity, the cookbook is designed to enable you reclaim control over your nutritional intake and enjoy a fulfilling and satisfying culinary experience.

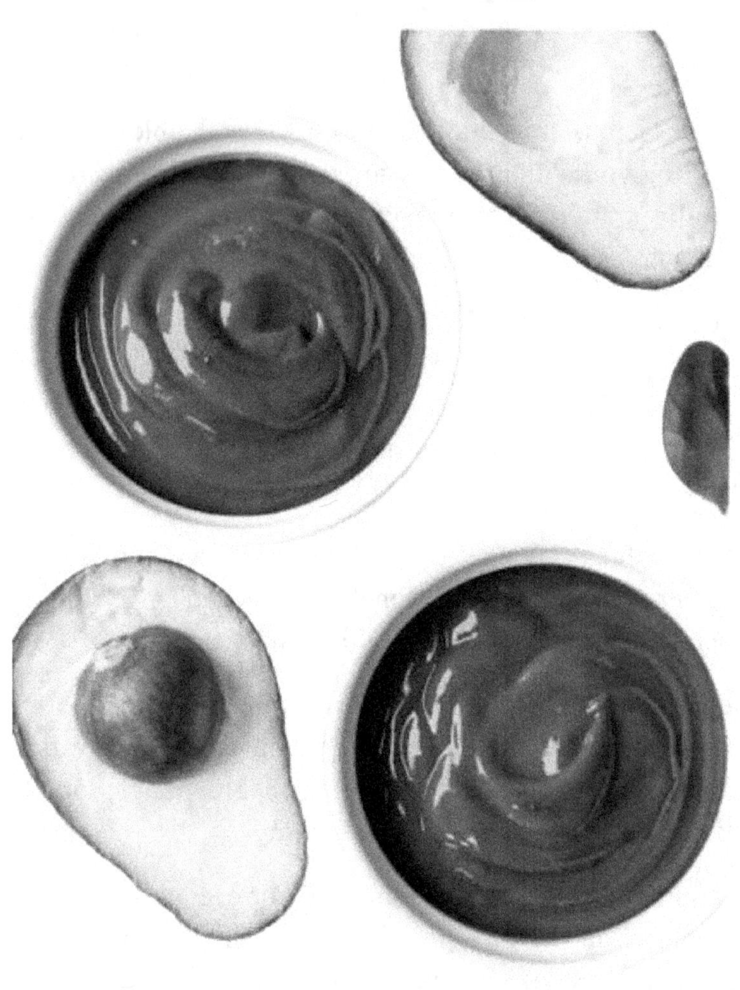

www.ingramcontent.com/pod-product-compliance
Lightning Source LLC
Chambersburg PA
CBHW050811250726
48653CB00006B/2170